OVERCOME INSOMNIA & WAKE UP HAPPY EVERY DAY

5 Bulletproof Secrets to Sleep Smarter, Relax and Fall Asleep Fast Every Night (Guaranteed Stress Relief!)

Adam Walker & Alexis Matthew

errors, omissions, or inaccuracies.

TABLE OF CONTENTS

CHAPTER 1:
INTRODUCTION
TYPES OF INSOMNIA

Do you struggle every night when trying to fall asleep?

Do you frequently wake up at night and spend countless hours awake in bed?

If you've ever suffered from Insomnia, you're about to get an accelerated course on what causes it and how to deal with it.

There are three types of Insomnia:

Type 1 Sleep Onset Insomnia

You cannot go to sleep and have to lie in bed between 30 minutes and 4 hours(or more) before you finally fall asleep, after quite a lot of stress, tossing and turning.

You usually wake up with a massive headache, feeling drowsy, or with your whole body aching.

Type 2 Sleep Maintenance Insomnia

You manage to go to sleep normally, but you wake up several times during the night and can't go back to sleep, or it takes you a long time to do so.

Type 3 Sleep Disturbance Insomnia

You go to sleep normally, you sleep for a normal amount of time (7-8 hours for adults, 5-6 hours for the elderly), but you wake up feeling unrested, with a headache, or feeling drowsy or dizzy.

Most Insomniacs find themselves suffering from a combination of type 1 and 2.

Type 3 is usually provoked by Sleep Apnea or PLM (periodic limb movement), or other underlying sleep disorders.

During pregnancy it is very common to experience type 3 Insomnia, especially in the last three to six months.

What you'll discover today is that there's a very interesting mechanism that actually prevents people with insomnia from sleeping!

First of all we have to distinguish between short-term insomnia and chronic Insomnia.

Short term Insomnia IS quite common and linked to natural occurrences in our lives, stress level or family and relationship problems.

Everyone suffers from it at some point, for example depression and other various health problems are very common to cause Insomnia.

The thing is, for most people short term Insomnia only lasts a few days before returning to their normal sleep patterns.

But for some unfortunate other, short term Insomnia never ends, becoming a part of their lives and turning into Chronic Insomnia.

Chronic Insomnia happens when you have regular long term sleeping problems.

Falling asleep now feels like a chore: drowsiness, headaches, depression, and low energy are your bread and butter.

I've been there, I know how it feels.

It's terrible and it's time to put a stop to it.

Now I want to ask you, what's the difference between someone with sleeping problems and someone who can fall asleep easily?

The answer lies in the natural sleep response.

Our sleep is divided in 4 stages. During stage 1 our brain waves lower from beta waves to alpha and theta waves, and we enter a dream stage that takes us deeper and deeper into sleep.

This is an automatic and natural response for most people and it happens after lying in bed for a few minutes. The moment we lay our head on our pillow and close our eyes, our brain gets a signal saying: "Alright, this is it. It's sleep time, let's lower the heart rate, the brain waves and fall asleep!".

When the natural sleep response doesn't work right, Chronic Insomnia happens.

In the most severe cases, the natural sleep response might be completely deleted, this phenomenon is called "negative anchor" and it leads to Chronic Insomnia.

Insomnia is often times linked to a lifestyle of bad sleeping habits that leads to very unfulfilling sleep.

Like most people, at some point in your life you probably experienced some short term Insomnia.

Something happened, you couldn't sleep, maybe for a few days or weeks.

What is stopping us from getting good sleep? How can we fight short term Insomnia?

As you can imagine, short term Insomnia too is provoked by a disruption of our natural sleep response.

We are unable to enter Stage 1 sleep, we are laying in bed and our brain waves stay in beta brain wave range, not allowing us to fall asleep.

CHAPTER 2:
AN OVERLY ACTIVE MIND

Picture this, you are lying in bed, wide awake, and you can't sleep because your mind just won't stop thinking and rest.

If this is a familiar scenario, I'm sorry to break it to you but an active mind has nothing to do with your inability to sleep.

It's actually quite the opposite, being awake makes your mind wander and think.

Let me explain this a little bit better: our thoughts work similarly to a snowball that's rolling down a hill. The snow ball gradually gets bigger and bigger and bigger gaining momentum and so do our thoughts.

The moment you apply focus to a single thought, you are going to keep thinking about it and that's going to lead you to more and more connected thoughts.

Did this make any sense to you?

Let's try a simple experiment, don't do any of the following.

DON'T picture a blue ice cream truck driving down a long road with trees on both sides.

Let me guess, you pictured what I just asked you not to, did you?

Our mind works by continuously taking in data and processing it.

This process is almost entirely out of your control and that's fine.

You cannot NOT think about a bright blue ice cream truck because whenever I mention it your mind has to picture an ice cream truck mini van to even think about it.

It's almost like our brain has a "mind of its own" and it will move in directions without you being even aware of it.

If your thoughts require too much conscious thinking, the amount of brain power needed for them will prevent you from entering Stage 1 Sleep.

Most of us are conditioned to just think about nothing when we go to sleep, our mind naturally just shuts off after a while and we go into Stage 1 sleep.

During stressful times though, our thoughts and focus change their flow and tend to take very un sleepy directions.

Our thoughts can easily turn from a walk in a park to re living stressful situations over and over again, simply because of this momentum concept.

What can you do to stop this?

Simple: don't try to FORCE sleep to come, rather just focus your attention on relaxing your body and mind.

Focus your imagination on pleasant, enjoyable and natural thoughts you don't need much effort to evocate.

Otherwise you will get stuck in a vicious cycle: the more you focus on trying to fall asleep the more you won't be able to, increasing your frustration.

Relaxing your body and mind lowers your brain waves and as you know by now, low brain waves are the gateway to Stage 1 Sleep.

Another big reason why a lot of people struggle with relaxing once they go to bed is because they engage in very mind stimulating activities such as discussing or arguing with others or working on their computer.

A wind down period of at least 45 minutes is always needed before you go to bed.

Meditation is of great help and I strongly suggest looking into it, even just 10 minutes a day can make a huge difference.

CHAPTER 3:
DOES COUNTING SHEEP ACTUALLY WORKS?

When you think about it, an army of sheep jumping over a fence isn't exactly the most calming scenario ever, so why are you forcing your mind to picture it in order to relax?

On top of that, sheep are INCREDIBLY lazy animals, you'd be better off counting them as they sleep on a peaceful green meadow.

Try this instead.

THE SLOW METHOD

works incredibly well, all you have to do is try to hear or visualize your thoughts as if you were saying them out loud or writing them down on a piece of paper and start consciously

slowing

them

down.

Play them in slow motion!

Keep replaying the same thought slower and slower, over and over again, shortening it every time until it fades completely.

This method works for two reasons:

1) It makes your mind distract from your inability to sleep and frustration;

2) It drives your thoughts into a positive direction and it focuses your mind on relaxing thoughts.

There will be a little resistance from your mind at the start and you will get distracted by random thoughts racing into your mind, but keep going and trying and you will find yourself asleep before you even realise what's happening!

THE CHALKBOARD METHOD

does wonders if you are a highly visual person.

As soon as your mind starts racing, try to visualise your thoughts as if they were being written on a blackboard at the same time as the new thoughts arrive.

Let's take this phrase as an example:

"Hmmm what am I going to wear tomorrow?"

When you have your sentence on the chalkboard, visualize yourself slowly wiping the phrase off it, leaving nothing but a blank chalkboard there.

The concept behind this method is the same as the previous one, try it out and let me know how it goes.

CHAPTER 4:
SET RULES AND RESTRICTIONS

This is perhaps the most powerful technique you will find out there to battle Insomnia.

Make up rules to follow when trying to fall asleep: if you can't fall asleep after lying in bed for more than 30 minutes, get out of bed!

Stay out until you feel your body getting sleepy and drowsy and only then go back to bed.

You might be skeptical about this, but it really works!

Your pattern of thinking gets suddenly interrupted the

moment you get out of bed.

If your mind was racing on its own, the chances that it will just suddenly stop while you keep doing exactly what you were doing before are incredibly low.

All of that negative momentum you created is keeping you awake and it must be interrupted at all cost.

Simply getting out of bed is an incredibly effective way to clear up your mind and it will help you restore your bed associations.

What are bed associations?

Let me give you a scenario first and see if this has ever happened to you.

It's the end of the day and you are tired, you're yawning and you can't wait to go to bed and get some rest.

You put on your pajamas, turn off the lights, get into bed… and suddenly you're wide awake and you don't feel tired at all.

How could this happen?

Well, fear not, this is way more common than you would think and it has a lot to do with your bed associations.

Our mind links experiences to emotions or states of mind, it's automatic and it happens unconsciously.

This process in hypnosis is known as anchoring.

An anchor is an experience, a feeling, it could be a taste, a smell or a sound that immediately recreates an emotional state in your body by association.

You have most definitely had it happen with certain songs that bring up specific memories or feelings every time you hear them.

Your bed is no exception: if you tend to watch TV in bed a lot, or read to try induce sleepiness, I have some bad news for you, you are not making your insomnia any better.

These actions not only keep your mind awake, they also anchor feelings associated to being awake to your bed.

This will trick your brain into thinking that your bed is a place where it has to be active.

This completely disturbs the natural sleep response.

Your bed should ONLY be used for sleeping and sexual activity, nothing else.

In an ideal world, you would use your bedroom just to sleep, while you workout, study or work in other areas of the house but that's not always possible.

Still, try to do your best and avoid any distracting activity in the evening or during the day in your bedroom.

CHAPTER 5:
THE IMPACT OF YOUR BODY TEMPERATURE

If your body temperature is not dropping at night might be one of the reasons why you are having trouble falling asleep.

This could mean a couple different things: either you are not getting enough sunlight or exercise during the day or simply you need less sleep to function and your body is signaling it to you.

A good trick is to take a hot shower before bed, if done correctly it will help you drop your body temperature.

In order for it to work, the bath or shower must be taken 60 to 90 minutes before going to sleep, not less.

A hot shower makes your body temperature rise quickly, which is why a hot shower in the morning is so refreshing.

After about 60 minutes though, your body temperature will start dropping, which is also why we feel so sluggish in the morning for the first hour after waking up (a short workout is a good remedy to that and it's definitely a lot healthier than caffeine).

If you try to sleep right after a hot shower, your high body temperature will actually make it quite difficult to fall asleep.

A drop in body temperature is a natural trigger for your brain that will send a signal to your muscles, telling them to relax as the brain waves get lower and lower until you enter stage 1 sleep.

Your own room's temperature is also something you should not underestimate as it directly affects your sleep quality on top of your ability to fall asleep.

If you sleep in a very hot or humid environment, you will have trouble sleeping deeply as the heat won't allow your body to lower its temperature.

Studies show that falling asleep in a cool room is much easier than falling asleep in a hot environment.

You also sleep more deeply when you're in a cool environment.

It goes without saying that you should not exaggerate as freezing won't help you sleep either!

As a small note since we are on the topic, I'd like to point out that light has a big impact on your sleep too as our body can produce melatonin only in complete darkness.

Melatonin is a hormone that regulates our sleep and the more melatonin is in your body, the easier it is to fall asleep.

If you have too much light in your room while you sleep, your melatonin levels will be affected so make sure you sleep in the dark!

CHAPTER 6:
SLEEPING PILLS
A TERRIBLE SOLUTION

Sleeping pills are bad.

In fact they are so bad that they often turn short term Insomnia into Chronic Insomnia.ia.

Throughout the 19th century the only sleeping pills available were Barbiturates (you might have heard of them as Marilyn Monroe died of overdosing on them).

Just about 10 of them was enough to cause an overdose.

Things have changed now but sleeping pills are still dangerous tools that should be only used in extreme situations and with caution.

There are 4 types available:

1) Benzodiazepines

2) Antidepressants

3) Over the Counter Drugs

4) Synthetic Melatonin

We will not go over the details of how these pills work, and the side effects of each one as it would go beyond the scope of this book.

Sure they may put a person to sleep but at what price!

The amount of side effects and chemicals they put in your body is insane and they can stay in your blood for up to 6 days!

Just to mention some, the side effects of these chemicals are often daytime drowsiness, nausea, blurred vision, weakness, loss of appetite, and in some cases very frequent urination.

The National Institute of Health advices that sleeping pills should not be prescribed to a patient for more than 4 to 6 weeks to make sure that the body doesn't get too accustomed to them, causing addiction.

The problem is that some doctors actually prescribe them for MONTHS or even YEARS.

Sleeping pills are not a final cure, Insomnia is not a disease or sickness that has to be cured with medicines, it's an inner system that you can correct once you know the mechanics of it.

Prescribing sleeping pills is just a lazy way to avoid dealing with a patient's problems directly and, as doctors receive quite poor training on sleeping problems, prescribing these pills is an easy solution for them.

The price patients will pay in the long run is huge as they often become completely dependant on them both physically and psychologically, making their lives even more miserable.

Most sleeping pills work by depressing the activity of the brain, and forcing lower brain waves.

Because of the nature of how sleeping pills work, they deprive you of deep sleep, making the actual sleep's quality terrible.

A study by Dr. Daniel F. Kripke of the University of California shows that people who use sleeping pills regularly have a much higher mortality (death) rate than people who don't.

If you are using sleeping pills, do yourself a favor and stop.

Oh and also, NEVER mix sleeping pills with alcohol.

CONCLUSION

Insomnia is demonized and looked at as a problem to solve.

In reality it is a symptom of a weak and damaged sleeping system.

Fixing your sleeping habits and strengthening your sleeping system by using the methods I illustrated in this book will do wonders.

If someone has a weak sleep system it is very difficult for that person to sleep deeply, therefore they experience a lot more Stage 2 sleep, and awakenings are even more likely to happen.

Break this endless loop of misery and improve your life now.

Try out these tricks and get your well deserved energy and happiness back!

Best of luck and goodnight.

45

ACKNOWLEDGEMENTS

The purpose of this book is to make your life better by improving your sleep quality and help you finally get rid of insomnia and any other common sleep disorder.

We want to thank you for taking action by reading this book and we hope that you keep on using these simple and efficient methods in order to reach your goal.
If you found this helpful, we hope that you can spread the word to everyone around you who struggles with the same problems in order to help them.

We also want to thank all of the members of our publishing team for making this possible.

A special thanks goes also to all of the researchers who study this matter every day at the cost of their own sleep to help us improve our nights and days.

Thank you all.